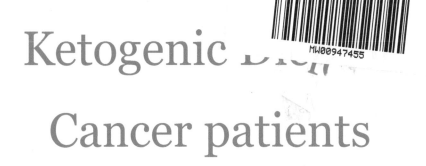

Ketogenic Diet

Cancer patients

Essential Guide to fight Cancer with Low
carbs, Fat burns, and Metabolic Nutrition's

Dr. Jemy Cole

Table of Contents

Introduction

Few struggles are as difficult and agonizing as the war against cancer in the broad field of human perseverance and fortitude. Each person who faces this tremendous foe sets out on a path that is very personal and is distinguished by unflinching resolve and an unquenchable desire to succeed. The ketogenic diet has emerged as a ray of hope among the many tactics used by cancer patients to help them battle the disease. The ketogenic diet, which was first developed to treat epilepsy, has drawn interest for its potential to help cancer patients fight this life-threatening disease. The ketogenic diet is examined in this article along with its physiological effects and potential benefits for people dealing with cancer.

A Ketogenic Diet: What Is It?

The ketogenic diet is a high-fat, low-carb eating plan that places an emphasis on cutting back significantly on your intake of carbohydrates while upping your intake of fats and keeping your protein intake in check. This dietary strategy aims to cause the metabolic state of ketosis, which is usually triggered by a severe carbohydrate restriction and occurs when the body primarily uses ketone bodies for energy instead of glucose.

A Ketogenic Diet: How Does It Operate?

The primary energy source for the human body is glucose, which is made from carbs. However, the body switches to burning fat reserves for energy when carbohydrate consumption is substantially reduced. Ketones, which the liver produces from fats during this process, replace glucose as the main energy source for the body and brain. The ketosis state is characterized by this change in metabolism.

The body's insulin levels fall during a ketogenic state, promoting the conversion of stored fat into fatty acids and the subsequent creation of ketones. Cells, particularly the brain, which generally relies largely on glucose, can then use these ketones for energy. The ensuing rise in ketone levels promotes a more steady and long-lasting energy source, possibly providing a number of advantages.

Why Could a Ketogenic Diet Help Patients with Cancer?

The Warburg effect, which occurs when cancer cells depend more heavily than normal on glucose for energy, has been demonstrated through research. This distinctive metabolic preference serves as the foundation for research into the ketogenic diet's potential as a cancer adjuvant therapy.

Starving Cancer Cells: The ketogenic diet tries to starve cancer cells and prevent their development and multiplication by substantially reducing carbohydrate intake and so restricting the availability of glucose.

Enhancing Cellular Stress Resistance: It has been discovered that ketones increase the resilience of normal cells to stress, while potentially weakening and rendering more vulnerable cancer cells.

Ketogenic diets have been connected to decreased inflammation, which has been linked to the development and progression of cancer.

Normalizing Insulin Levels: Because high insulin levels have been linked to the proliferation of specific cancer cells, a ketogenic diet may help manage insulin levels, which can be helpful for cancer patients.

Improving Weight Management: Certain cancers might be increased by obesity and excess body fat. The ketogenic diet can help with fat loss and weight management, which may benefit cancer patients' prognoses.

The ketogenic diet presents itself as a potential addition to traditional cancer treatments, while research in this area is still underway. It is essential for people thinking about this dietary approach to speak with medical professionals and customize the diet to their unique needs and circumstances. Every feasible route for assistance and recovery should be investigated and taken into consideration because the fight against cancer is never-ending.

Ketogenic Diet Side Effects and Potential Risks

While some people may benefit from the ketogenic diet, it's important to recognize that, like any dietary strategy, it has possible hazards and adverse effects. Making decisions about implementing a ketogenic diet should be done with knowledge of these factors in mind.

1. Keto Flu: During the initial shift into ketosis, people may have signs and symptoms like the flu, such as exhaustion, headaches, nausea, and irritability.

Cause: This happens as the body gets used to using ketones as its primary energy source rather than glucose.

2. Electrolyte Imbalance: Due to increased urine and reduced intake of specific foods, a ketogenic diet can result in a loss of electrolytes such salt, potassium, and magnesium.

Effect: Electrolyte imbalances can result in weariness, weakness, and, in extreme situations, heart problems.

3. Nutrient Deficiencies: Limiting some food groups may cause an insufficient intake of vital nutrients like vitamins, minerals, and fiber.

Effect: Prolonged vitamin deficiency can impair the nutritional balance and cause health problems.

4. Digestive Problems: When changing to a high-fat, low-carbohydrate diet, some people may develop constipation or diarrhea.

Cause: Dietary changes that alter the gut flora and fiber intake can be a factor in gastrointestinal pain.

5. Potential Impact on Cholesterol Levels: Summary: For some people, the ketogenic diet may result in a rise in LDL cholesterol, sometimes known as "bad" cholesterol.

Monitoring: It's important to keep an eye on your cholesterol levels, especially if you already have heart disease.

6. Negative Effect on Athletic Performance: During the initial phase of adjusting to ketosis, athletes taking part in demanding, endurance-based activities may see a decline in performance.

Reason: Ketones might not supply enough energy for some high-intensity exercises.

Who Should Consult a Physician Before Beginning a Ketogenic Diet?

The ketogenic diet isn't right for everyone, so some people should speak with a doctor before starting it to be sure it's safe and acceptable for them.

1. People who already have a major medical condition, such as diabetes, liver disease, renal illness, heart disease, pancreatitis, or any other ailment.

neurological conditions other than epilepsy, as the effects of the diet can change depending on the particular ailment.

2. Women who are expecting or nursing: It is important to carefully consider the potential consequences of a ketogenic diet on both the mother and the unborn child.

3. People who take drugs: Due to the changed metabolic state brought on by a ketogenic diet, several medications may need to be adjusted.

4. People with a History of Eating Disorders: People with a history of disordered eating should follow any restrictive diet under close supervision, including the ketogenic diet.

5. Young Children: To promote proper growth and development, the ketogenic diet for epileptic children needs specific medical supervision and monitoring.

6. Individuals with a history of gallbladder problems: High-fat diets may make gallbladder issues worse, thus they should be avoided and under medical supervision.

It is critical to get medical advice before beginning a ketogenic diet, especially for people with pre-existing diseases or unique circumstances. The ketogenic diet can be followed safely and efficiently, limiting potential hazards and optimizing potential benefits, with the help of a comprehensive evaluation and the right supervision.

How to Begin the Ketogenic Diet?

The low-carb, high-fat, and moderate-protein ketogenic diet has grown in popularity because of its possible health advantages. Following a well-planned ketogenic diet can have many positive effects, but in order to enter and stay in ketosis, it's important to know which items to eat and which to avoid.

What to Eat on a Ketogenic Diet:

Healthy Fats:

Avocados: Full of fiber and good fats.

MCTs (medium-chain triglycerides) are abundant in coconut oil.

A good source of monounsaturated fats is olive oil.

Low-carb healthy fats like butter and ghee.

Proteins:

Choose high-quality, unprocessed meats like beef, chicken, and fish while eating.

Eggs are a key component of the ketogenic diet and a flexible source of protein.

Fish: Omega-3 fatty acids are abundant in fatty fish like salmon and mackerel.

Nuts and Seeds: Excellent choices include almonds, chia seeds, flaxseeds, and walnuts.

Low-Carb Produce:

Spinach, kale, lettuce, and other leafy greens are low in carbohydrates.

Cruciferous Vegetables: Brussels sprouts, cauliflower, and broccoli are all acceptable keto food choices.

Adding variety to your meals with low-carb options like bell peppers, zucchini, and asparagus.

Dairy:

Pick unprocessed cheeses such cream cheese, mozzarella, and cheddar.

Greek yogurt is low in carbs and high in protein.

Berries:

Blueberries, raspberries, and strawberries Compared to other fruits, they have fewer carbs.

Sweeteners:

Keto-friendly sweeteners with little effect on blood sugar levels include stevia, erythritol, and xylitol.

Beverages:

Water: It's important to stay hydrated.

Unsweetened and without milk for coffee and tea.

What to Stay Away From While on a Ketogenic Diet

High-Carb Foods:

grains: oats, wheat, rice, and other types of grains.

Sugars: All added sugars, such as those found in candy, sweets, and sugar-sweetened beverages.

Fruits: Fruits with a lot of sugar, such as bananas, apples, and oranges.

Veggies That Are Starchy:

Sweet potatoes, corn, and potatoes are all high in carbs and should be avoided.

Finished Products:

Bread, crackers, chips, and cookies: high in carbohydrates and frequently contain bad fats.

Sweet Condiments

Honey, syrups, and ketchup are all high in sugar and carbs.

Sauces with more sugar:

Sauces like barbecue, teriyaki, and sweetened salad dressings are frequently loaded with unrecognized sugars.

Sugary dairy products:

Ice cream, flavor-infused milk, and sweetened yogurt all have extra sugars.

Beans and legumes:

High in carbs are kidney beans, chickpeas, and lentils.

A ketogenic diet requires a change in eating habits that places a greater emphasis on wholesome fats, enough protein, and little carbohydrates. Before making significant dietary changes, always get the advice of a medical practitioner or a trained dietitian to be sure they are in line with your needs and health objectives.

Meal preparation and ketogenic diet recipes

Planning meals carefully is necessary when following a ketogenic diet in order to ensure appropriate nourishment and maintain the macronutrient ratios required for ketosis. Here is a guide to assist you in creating a ketogenic diet meal plan and some sample recipes.

Tips for Meal Planning: Balance Macronutrients

To get a daily macronutrient ratio of roughly 70–80% fats, 15–25% protein, and 5–10% carbohydrates, use the following table.

Including Healthy Fats

To get your recommended daily intake of fat, choose foods like avocados, olive oil, nuts, seeds, and oily salmon.

Moderate Protein Included:

Choose lean proteins such tofu and tempeh, as well as fish, eggs, and fish.

Pick Low-Carb Veggies:

To limit your intake of carbohydrates, include non-starchy veggies like spinach, broccoli, zucchini, and cauliflower.

Plan your desserts and snacks carefully:

Choose sweets with sweeteners that are permitted for the keto diet, as well as keto-friendly snacks like nuts, cheese, or berries.

Sample recipes for a ketogenic diet

Avocado and egg breakfast bowl for keto

Avocado, eggs, cherry tomatoes, spinach, salt, pepper, and olive oil are the ingredients.

Prepare eggs according to your choice, then top with cherry tomatoes and sautéed spinach.

Chicken and broccoli salad for a keto lunch.

Grilled chicken, broccoli, olive oil, lemon juice, salt, pepper, and Parmesan cheese are the ingredients.

Instructions: Add olive oil, lemon juice, and Parmesan cheese to the grilled chicken and steamed broccoli before serving.

Dinner on the keto diet: salmon with cauliflower mash and asparagus

Salmon fillet, asparagus, cauliflower, butter, garlic, salt, and pepper are the ingredients.

Instructions: Steam cauliflower, mash with butter, and season with garlic, salt, and pepper. Bake salmon and asparagus.

Low-carb Snack: Fat Bombs

Cream cheese, coconut oil, cocoa powder, stevia, and chopped nuts are the ingredients.

Instructions: Combine the cream cheese, chocolate powder, stevia, and coconut oil. Make into balls, sprinkle with chopped nuts, and chill.

Supplements that Cancer Patients on a Ketogenic Diet May Find Beneficial

Cancer patients may benefit from the ketogenic diet, but supplementation must be done carefully and with a doctor's approval. The following supplements can be taken into consideration after seeing a doctor:

fatty acids omega-3

Omega-3s, which are present in fish oil supplements, help promote heart health and lessen inflammation.

the vitamin D

essential for immunological wellness and bone health. Low levels are common in cancer patients, who may profit from supplementation.

Electrolytes:

It may be advised to take supplements like magnesium, potassium, and sodium due to probable electrolyte imbalances on a ketogenic diet.

Minerals and multivitamins:

to fill in any nutrient deficiencies that may exist in the diet, especially if the variety and consumption of vegetables are restricted.

Medium-Chain Triglycerides, or MCT Oil:

MCT oil, a source of easily accessible ketones, can help achieve and sustain ketosis.

Supplements with protein:

for people who have trouble getting enough protein from food alone, especially if they are receiving therapy for an ailment that affects their appetite or digestion.

Consult your medical team before incorporating any supplements into your routine to make sure they are secure and suitable for your unique situation, state of health, and ongoing therapies. The ketogenic diet can be complemented by a targeted approach to supplementation, which can help create an all-encompassing treatment strategy for cancer patients.

Managing the Side Effects of Cancer Treatment with the Ketogenic Diet

Cancer therapies like chemotherapy and radiation frequently have a variety of unpleasant side effects. The ketogenic diet has been investigated as a supportive therapy to control these adverse effects while receiving cancer treatment due to its capacity to normalize blood sugar levels and decrease inflammation. Here's a discussion on how the ketogenic diet may help with some particular adverse effects of treatment.

1. Tiredness

A frequent side effect of cancer treatment is fatigue, which can be brought on by the illness itself or other factors like anemia, poor diet, or interrupted sleep cycles. The ketogenic diet may aid in the management of fatigue by:

Stabilizing Energy Levels: By lowering blood sugar variations, the ketogenic diet can offer a stable and prolonged supply of energy, potentially assisting in the fight against exhaustion brought on by glucose spikes and crashes.

Ketones, the main fuel source on a ketogenic diet, are effectively used by mitochondria, boosting cellular energy output and possibly lowering fatigue.

Anti-Inflammatory Effects: The anti-inflammatory effects of the ketogenic diet may help lessen fatigue brought on by inflammation, which is frequently experienced after cancer therapies.

2. Vomiting and Nausea

The unpleasant side effects of cancer therapies, especially chemotherapy, include nausea and vomiting. The ketogenic diet might provide comfort by

Blood Sugar Stabilization: The ketogenic diet can aid in blood sugar stabilization, potentially lowering instances of nausea brought on by blood sugar variations.

Reducing Sugar Intake: Since sugar can occasionally make nausea worse, reducing sugar intake, a feature of the ketogenic diet, may help

Giving the Digestive System a Rest: Ketogenic meals' ease of preparation and ease of digestion may help to reduce gastrointestinal discomfort, including nausea and vomiting.

3. vomiting and diarrhea

One typical gastrointestinal adverse effect of cancer treatment is diarrhea. The ketogenic diet may aid in the management of diarrhea by:

Maintaining a healthy gut microbiota can help prevent diarrhea if a ketogenic diet is properly prepared and includes enough fiber from low-carb veggies.

Avoiding Trigger meals: The ketogenic diet may offer relief by avoiding high-carb, sugary, and processed meals that might aggravate diarrhea.

The ketogenic diet places a strong emphasis on drinking more water, which can help prevent dehydration, a danger that is connected to diarrhea.

4. indigestion

Another digestive problem that cancer patients frequently experience is constipation, which could be brought on by drugs, a decline in activity level, or dietary modifications. The ketogenic diet may help with constipation management by

Increasing Fiber Intake: Although the ketogenic diet has a low overall carbohydrate intake, low-carb, fiber-rich vegetables can still be included. These vegetables may assist regular bowel movements and relieve constipation.

Water intake should be increased as recommended by the ketogenic diet in order to maintain regular bowel movements and avoid constipation.

Electrolyte Balance: The ketogenic diet places an emphasis on maintaining proper electrolyte balance, which can improve overall gut health and relieve constipation.

Before making big dietary changes, such as switching to a ketogenic diet, it's crucial to speak with a doctor to make sure they are in line with your treatment plan and cater to your individual needs and concerns. To guarantee that it improves overall wellness and aids cancer therapy, the ketogenic diet should be tailored to the individual and closely monitored.

How to Use the Ketogenic Diet to Overcome Cancer-Related Obstacles?

Numerous difficulties are frequently brought on by cancer and its therapies, which have an effect on the general wellbeing of those who are afflicted. It is being investigated as a potential solution to some of these problems to use the ketogenic diet, which is well known for its potential advantages in treating a number of medical disorders. This article explores how the ketogenic diet can help with the weight loss, cachexia, discomfort, and neuropathy that are frequently felt by cancer patients.

Losing weight

Cancer patients frequently worry about losing weight, which is frequently ascribed to a variety of factors, such as metabolic changes, decreased appetite, and the body's increased energy requirements during cancer therapy. The following ways the ketogenic diet may aid with weight management:

The ketogenic diet promotes the body to utilise fat that has been stored as energy, which may help with weight loss while protecting lean body mass.

Ketones, which are created during ketosis, have been linked to suppressed hunger, which may be helpful for people who are having trouble maintaining a healthy weight.

Blood Sugar Stabilization: The ketogenic diet aids in blood sugar stabilization, which may lessen cravings and encourage a more regular, controlled eating habit.

Cachexia

Cancer patients frequently experience cachexia, a severe wasting illness marked by considerable weight loss, muscle atrophy, and exhaustion. Although additional research is required, the ketogenic diet may help to treat cachexia by

Maintaining Lean Muscle Mass: The ketogenic diet may lessen muscle atrophy by giving priority to burning fat over the breakdown of muscle.

Providing a Satisfying Diet: The ketogenic diet, with its emphasis on protein and good fats, may aid people in feeling satisfied for a longer period of time, meeting their dietary requirements.

Pain

Pain brought on by cancer can be crippling and impair one's quality of life. Although the ketogenic diet is not a method for directly managing pain, it may nonetheless have an indirect impact on how pain is perceived and managed by

Reducing Inflammation: The ketogenic diet has anti-inflammatory properties that may help reduce pain brought on by inflammation.

Weight loss accomplished by the ketogenic diet can ease joint tension and may even lessen pain in people who are experiencing musculoskeletal discomfort.

Neuritis

Chemotherapy frequently results in neuropathy, which causes pain, numbness, and tingling in the extremities. Although the ketogenic diet cannot treat neuropathy, it may aid with symptom management by

Stabilizing Blood Sugar Levels: The ketogenic diet may lessen nerve damage brought on by blood sugar swings by maintaining stable blood sugar levels.

reducing inflammation: The ketogenic diet's anti-inflammatory effects could help with neuropathic pain brought on by inflammation.

Before beginning a ketogenic diet, especially while receiving treatment for cancer, it is imperative to speak with a healthcare provider, especially a qualified dietitian or nutritionist. They can modify the diet to meet specific demands, ensuring that it promotes general health and works in tandem with the continuing cancer management strategy. To effectively address the difficulties faced by cancer patients, a multidisciplinary strategy that includes medical monitoring, dietary modifications, and pain management techniques is essential.

Ketogenic Diet and the Treatment

of Cancer

The ketogenic diet, known for its high-fat, low-carbohydrate composition, has drawn interest recently due to its potential to aid in the treatment of cancer. For those considering include the ketogenic diet in their cancer management strategy, it is crucial to comprehend how it may interact with conventional cancer therapies including chemotherapy, radiation therapy, and immunotherapy.

1. The impact of chemotherapy

Chemotherapy is a popular cancer treatment that tries to eradicate cancer cells that divide quickly. The ketogenic diet and chemotherapy may interact as follows:

Potential Synergistic Effect: According to some research, combining a ketogenic diet with chemotherapy may increase the latter's effectiveness, perhaps resulting in higher rates of tumor regression and better treatment results.

Metabolic Sensitization: By modifying the tumor microenvironment and making cancer cells more vulnerable to the harmful effects of some chemotherapy drugs, the ketogenic diet may make cancer cells more sensitive to the effects of chemotherapy.

Reduced negative Effects: By offering a more consistent and long-lasting energy supply, the ketogenic diet may help reduce some negative effects of chemotherapy, such as weariness.

2. Radiation Therapy Interaction

High-energy particles or waves are used in radiation therapy to kill or harm cancer cells. According to the following, radiation therapy and the ketogenic diet may interact:

Enhanced Sensitivity of Cancer Cells: According to some studies, the ketogenic diet may make cancer cells more susceptible to radiation therapy, which could enhance the radiation's therapeutic benefits.

Healthy cells frequently adapt better to using ketones for energy than cancer cells, suggesting that the ketogenic diet may shield them from radiation-induced damage.

Reduced Inflammation: By lowering inflammation and oxidative stress in the body, the ketogenic diet may complement radiation therapy.

3. How Immunotherapy Reacts

In immunotherapy, cancer cells are targeted and eliminated by the body's immune system. The ketogenic diet may interact with immunotherapy in the following ways:

Effects on Immunomodulation: The ketogenic diet may have immunomodulatory properties that could work in concert with immunotherapy to improve the immune system's capacity to recognize and eliminate cancer cells.

Immune response balancing: By lowering chronic inflammation, which is frequently linked to cancer and may impair the effectiveness of immunotherapies, the ketogenic diet may help balance the immune response.

Maintaining Nutritional Status: If used correctly, the ketogenic diet can assist in ensuring appropriate nutrition during immunotherapy, which is essential for the immune system to perform at its best.

The use of the ketogenic diet as a complementary strategy to cancer treatment requires careful consideration and should be carried out with the help of healthcare professionals, despite the fact that there is still limited research on the possible synergy between the ketogenic diet and various cancer treatments. Based on a person's unique cancer type, stage, general health, and treatment objectives, individualized treatment programs that use the ketogenic diet should be created. To fully comprehend the breadth of interactions between the ketogenic diet and cancer therapy, additional research is required.

Dietary Ketosis and Cancer

Prognosis

Research and scientific study are being conducted to determine the potential effects of the ketogenic diet on cancer prognosis, including survival and recurrence rates. Here is a summary of what is known at this time based on the research that is available:

1. Ketogenic Diet and Survival from Cancer

The effects of the ketogenic diet on cancer survival are still being studied. Although some studies hint at potential advantages, more thorough and extensive research is required to reach definitive results. The following are some studies on the ketogenic diet and cancer survival:

Improved Metabolic Health: By stabilizing blood sugar levels and lowering inflammation, the ketogenic diet may favorably affect metabolic health, which may enhance general wellbeing during cancer treatment.

Enhanced Response to Treatment: Early-stage human and animal research suggests that the ketogenic diet may increase the efficacy of several cancer treatments, which may ultimately lead to higher survival rates.

Important Notes: It's crucial to keep in mind that the ketogenic diet shouldn't be used as a stand-alone cancer treatment. It should be considered as a potential supplementary therapy and carefully incorporated into a comprehensive treatment plan while being monitored by a doctor.

2. Cancer Recurrence with the Ketogenic Diet

Additionally, in its infancy, research on the ketogenic diet's impact on cancer recurrence has shown little results. More analysis and clinical trials are necessary to comprehend the ketogenic diet's possible effects on cancer recurrence. The following are some observations about the ketogenic diet and cancer recurrence:

Metabolic Alterations: The ketogenic diet alters the body's metabolism, possibly reducing the conditions that encourage the growth of cancer cells. This modification might affect the likelihood of a cancer recurrence, but more studies are required to confirm this.

Potential Anti-inflammatory benefits: Given that chronic inflammation is linked to cancer progression, the ketogenic diet's potential anti-inflammatory benefits may help lower the chance of cancer recurrence.

Individual Variability: Because cancer is such a complicated disease, each person's response to the ketogenic diet in terms of their risk of cancer recurrence will be unique. This response will depend on their particular cancer type, stage, genetics, and general state of health.

While there is growing evidence that the ketogenic diet may be helpful in the management of cancer, more thorough clinical trials and long-term studies are required to confirm its efficacy in impacting cancer survival and recurrence. To make sure it fits with their treatment plan and overall health, those who are thinking about using the ketogenic diet as part of their cancer management should do so in conjunction with their healthcare team. Finally, rather than serving as a replacement for current cancer treatments, the ketogenic diet may be used in addition to them.

Bonus: Ketogenic Diet for Particular Groups of Cancer Patients

Ketogenic Diet for Cancer in Children

Children with certain types of cancer, especially those with brain tumors, have benefited from the ketogenic diet. Health care specialists actively supervise the diet and carefully adjust it to each child's needs. Benefits could consist of:

Possible Tumor Growth Inhibition: According to some studies, some brain tumors may not grow as quickly when on the ketogenic diet.

Management of Seizures: The ketogenic diet, which was initially created to control epilepsy, may help decrease seizure frequency in children with brain tumors that are prone to generating seizures.

Nutritional Support: The ketogenic diet can supply the youngster with the calories and nutrients they need to grow and thrive while receiving cancer therapy.

The Ketogenic Diet for Seniors with Cancer

During therapy, elderly cancer patients frequently encounter particular difficulties. If followed properly, the ketogenic diet may provide the following advantages for this group:

Weight Control: The ketogenic diet may aid with weight control, which is crucial for elderly people who are coping with weakness and muscle loss.

The ketogenic diet may boost cognitive performance, which is important for the aged population, according to certain research.

Stabilized Blood Sugar Levels: Older people with diabetes or insulin resistance may benefit from the ketogenic diet's capacity to stabilize blood sugar levels.

Ketogenic Diet for Patients with Cancer and Other Medical Conditions

Aside from their cancer treatment, cancer patients frequently need to manage additional medical issues. These conditions can be accommodated by the ketogenic diet:

Diabetes: The ketogenic diet, which restricts carbohydrate intake, may help cancer patients with diabetes manage their blood sugar levels.

Cardiovascular Conditions: For cancer patients who have cardiovascular issues, careful fat selection in the ketogenic diet can be important, with a focus on heart-healthy alternatives.

Kidney illness: For cancer patients with kidney illness who are considering a ketogenic diet, adjustments to protein intake and monitoring of kidney function are crucial.

Recipes for Cancer Patients Who Are on the Ketogenic Diet

1. 2 cups of broccoli florets are required for the soup "Creamy Broccoli"

heavy cream, 1 cup

two cups of veggie broth and two tablespoons of butter.

pepper and salt as desired

grated cheddar cheese is optional as a garnish.

Directions: Sauté broccoli in butter in a pot for a few minutes.

When the broccoli is ready, add the vegetable broth and boil.

Blend the ingredients thoroughly.

Back in the pot, mix in the heavy cream, and slowly reheat.

Add salt and pepper to taste. If preferred, top with cheddar cheese and serve hot.

2. Salmon with Grilled Lemon and Garlic Ingredients: 4 salmon fillets

Olive oil, 4 tablespoons

2 minced garlic cloves with 1 lemon's zest and juice

pepper and salt as desired

garnishing with fresh parsley

To make a marinade, combine olive oil, garlic, lemon juice, and zest in a bowl.

Salmon fillets should be placed in a shallow dish, covered with the marinade, and allowed to marinate for 30 minutes.

Warm up the grill. Put some salt and pepper on the salmon.

Depending on how done you want your salmon, grill it for 5 to 7 minutes per side.

Before serving, garnish with fresh parsley.

Advice for Maintaining the Ketogenic Diet

Planning and preparing meals: To stay on the diet, prepare meals and snacks that are keto-friendly and plan your meals in advance.

Regular Monitoring: To make sure you're in ketosis and following the diet, keep an eye on your macronutrient ratios and overall carb intake.

Drink plenty of water to stay hydrated when following the ketogenic diet and to enhance your general wellbeing.

Include Variety: To keep your meals interesting and avoid diet fatigue, experiment with several keto-friendly items.

Seek Professional Guidance: For individualized advice and assistance, work closely with a registered dietitian or other healthcare professional with knowledge in ketogenic diets.

Always check with your medical team to be sure a diet is safe and suitable for your specific needs before beginning, especially if you are receiving treatment for cancer.

Conclusion

By affecting metabolism, inflammation, and other physiological processes, the ketogenic diet, which is characterized by its low-carbohydrate, high-fat composition, has shown promise in potentially assisting cancer patients. But it's essential to think of the ketogenic diet as an additional tactic within a thorough cancer treatment program.

Do You Need a Ketogenic Diet?

Your precise cancer type, stage, treatment plan, general health, and personal preferences will all play a role in determining whether the ketogenic diet is right for you. It's critical to speak with your medical team, which should include oncologists, dietitians, and other pertinent professionals, to ascertain whether the ketogenic diet is appropriate for your particular situation.

Considerations:

Cancer Type and Stage: Different types of cancer may react differently to dietary changes.

Address any underlying medical disorders that may affect the compatibility of the diet, such as diabetes or kidney problems.

Treatment Strategy Analyze the compatibility of the ketogenic diet with your ongoing and planned treatments.

Where to Go for More Support and Information

If you're interested in learning more about the ketogenic diet or in finding direction and support, take a look at the following resources:

Consult a Registered Dietitian: A Registered Dietitian with knowledge of both the ketogenic and cancer diets may offer you individualized suggestions and meal plans based on your unique requirements.

NCI: National Cancer Institute The NCI provides in-depth details on various cancer kinds, available treatments, and dietary considerations.

American Cancer Society (ACS): The ACS offers a multitude of materials, including details on cancer prevention, diagnosis, and treatment.

Ketogenic Diet Organizations and Websites: Research reliable sources for information about the ketogenic diet, such as the Charlie

Foundation (charliefoundation.org) and The Epilepsy Foundation (epilepsy.com).

Join local or online cancer support groups to meet others who have used the ketogenic diet to help them through their cancer journey.

Access scientific papers and publications to remain current on the most recent findings about the ketogenic diet and its possible application in the treatment of cancer.

The ketogenic diet may show potential as an additional treatment for some cancer patients, but each case should be examined separately. You can make an educated choice about the ketogenic diet's role in your cancer treatment and general well-being by working together with your healthcare team, acquiring facts from reliable sources, and taking into account your particular circumstances.

Made in United States
Troutdale, OR
01/07/2024

16770484R00030